Praise for

No One Runs Through My Garden Anymore

"If every parent and youth adopted just two or more of the healthy choices discussed in Hall's book, childhood obesity would quickly decline in this country."

– James P. Scibilia, MD,
Tri-State Pediatric Association

"No One Runs Through My Garden Anymore emphasizes that small steps over time are required to make significant changes in improving one's health. This uplifting story takes us back to basics and presents the obesity crisis (in both children and adults) in a captivating manner."

– Mary Alice Gettings,
Registered Dietitian and Certified Diabetes Educator

"This book illustrates the importance and positive impact of making children aware of all aspects of a healthy lifestyle."

– Darlene Farrell,
Family and Consumer Science Educator

No One Runs Through My Garden Anymore

One Boy's Quest to Beat Childhood Obesity by Getting Back to Nature

NO ONE RUNS THROUGH MY GARDEN ANYMORE

*One Boy's Quest to Beat Childhood
Obesity by Getting Back to Nature*

Roger Hall

No One Runs Through My Garden Anymore:
One Boy's Quest to Beat Childhood Obesity by Getting Back to Nature
© 2010
By Roger Hall

ISBN-13: 978-1453870914
ISBN: 1453870911

First Edition, 2010

Porcupine Communications, LLC,
PO Box 2338, Cranberry Township, PA 16066
www.porcupinecommunications.com

Cover Illustration – Amanda Joy Lee
Cover and Interior Design – Holly Rosborough Wensel,
Network Printing Services
Interior Illustrations – Bill Dotson
Editor – Gina Mazza

This book is for informational purposes only and is not intended to take the place of medical advice from healthcare professionals in your life. Readers are advised to consult with their medical doctor before undergoing any weight loss or healthcare regime.

10 9 8 7 6 5 4 3 2 1

DEDICATION

To God,
for the gift of life.

To nature,
for all its bounty.

To the animal world,
for its great wisdom.

To children everywhere,
may you experience the joy
of lifelong good health.

ACKNOWLEDGEMENTS

Many, many thanks to Gina Mazza, a brilliant writer
and health-conscious mother of two teenagers;
Nancy Brooks, for her strong business acumen; and
Darlene Farrell, for her helpful guidance in the creation
of the interactive exercises in this book.

Table of Contents

PART I:

❖

JASON'S STORY

CHAPTER ONE

THE CROW'S FATEFUL MESSAGE

Old Lady Thelma stood on the front porch of a farmhouse that she and her husband, William, called home for more than 50 years. Wistfully, she gazed at the fields they'd farmed for just as long. *I wonder why no one runs through my garden anymore,* she pondered.

Back in the day, kids of all ages would knock down her tomato plants and corn stalks as they took a short cut to the woods and pond beyond the fields. There, they would catch crawfish, cast a line for blue gills or skip rocks across the water. Sometimes, those same kids would frolic for hours right in the corn fields—playing hide and seek, and other childhood games.

Thelma turned to her grandson, Jason, who was sitting cross-legged on the porch. Jason was visiting his grandparent's farm in Pennsylvania during his New York State high school's spring break.

"How come nobody runs through my garden anymore?" she asked.

"What do you mean, Grandma?" he responded.

"I don't see kids your age outside anymore."

"Ah, we're too busy watching movies or TV shows on our portable laptops, I guess... or, playing games on our gaming devices, or chatting with friends on Internet social networking sites."

Thelma seethed inside upon hearing this. "Well, a report in the newspaper this morning said that kids are getting heavier and lazier, and it's because of just that: PCs and other types of portable technology that keep kids glued to screens!"

Just then, two lonely crows cawed in a distant field. Thelma knows a lot about nature—enough to know that crows are not songbirds but imitators of other sounds. In the wild, they imitate the shrill cry of the hawk and other birds of prey. And when crows see animals feasting on a carcass, they imitate the hawk's cry so the animals will flee and they can fly in for a private feast. Thelma also knows that crows often glide on the wind, and roll and dive at each other but they still have a mind of their own. They don't need to follow the wind—they go in their own direction.

As Thelma observed the crows in the field, it reminded her of a story she'd once heard about crows being kept in cages inside someone's home. In captivity, they imitated sounds like flushing toilets and tapping on a keyboard. Because they were fed fast food scraps, the crows grew obese and lethargic. Their feathers turned dull grey and fell out. Their beak colors faded. Eventually, they died and shriveled into what looked like lumps of fossilized coal at the bottom of the cage.

Was her dear grandson Jason going to suffer the same fate because of his techno-captive lifestyle and junk food diet? In the insular environment of home or school, kids can yell and scream but their voices are muffled by the synthetic materials all around. Over to the fridge then back to the TV...over to the desk then back to the computer keyboard. Over and back, tap, tap, tap, back and forth. The energy in such an environment becomes stuck, dull, uninspired.

It used to be that children playing on a wooded hillside

would frolic and holler, and nature would hear them. In response, trees would stand at attention like great sentinels. The wind would echo a refrain to each child's voice. Birds would fly close to see what was the matter. Even clouds would fly lower in response to their human brethren having so much fun. Mother Nature is always pleased to share her vibrant energy—especially with children—but where have all the little ones gone, she too wonders?

* * *

That night, Thelma had a bizarre dream about the crow story. It went like this: It was a hot summer evening and a violent thunderstorm clapped in the distance. The metal window shudders banged against the brick house, like death cracking its knuckles. The sounds even made the crows shiver in their cage. Then a flock of wild crows came in through the dryer vents to free their captive cousins. As their silhouettes reflected off the walls, the limp caged crows lifted their shriveled heads. The wild crows clawed into the cage and flung open its door with their beaks.

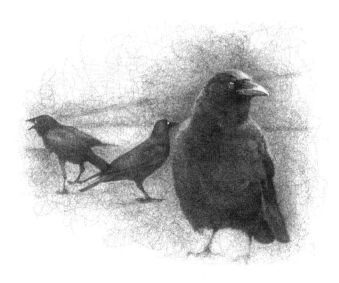

"Caw! Caw!" they shrieked, inciting the flaccid birds to follow them. The earthy scent of the wild crows' wet feathers—a delicious combination of evergreen and wildflower oils—revived the captive crows. They wanted to fly but were too heavy and weak. Just then, the crows' heads turned into those of Jason and his friends.

CHAPTER TWO

THELMA'S DREAM INTERPRETATION

The dream startled Thelma awake. Immediately, she knew the meaning behind it. Many kids today are not much different in their own electronic cages, imitating someone else's music, games or entertainment. They stay in artificial light and are mostly parked in front of the TV, the PC or portable music players where they imitate, not create. In fact, they are captive to high-speed electronic pipes and fiber optic cables. Learning effective communication goes by the wayside, as does original thinking. Their minds become fossilized—and so do their arteries from a diet of mostly processed foods.

Like anyone who's in tune with nature, Thelma knew that the way out of this unhealthy lifestyle was to "pull the plug" and get her grandchild back into the natural rhythm of things. She knows, for example, that every body of water on the planet (oceans, ponds, rivers, streams) has a built-in sundial that resets itself every day to be in synch with the sun, the moon, the clouds and weather patterns in the atmosphere. These bodies of water supply nutrients to all vegetation, the roots of trees worldwide and all animals.

All human beings have a sundial in their hearts, as well. We have to get outside everyday to reset this internal sundial and be in tune with nature. It also means being in tune with our internal drive to create and use our unique gifts; if not, the sundial rusts.

The next morning, Thelma shared her dream with Jason, and it really got him thinking about how much time he spends indoors, in front of an artificial screen. Jason loves his portable music player and computer paraphernalia but had to admit that something in him missed simple things like swinging upside down on the monkey bars at the local park and pulling carrots from the garden with Grandpa.

As Thelma walked to the kitchen to prepare a healthy break-fast for Jason—no toaster pastries today!—she once again noticed

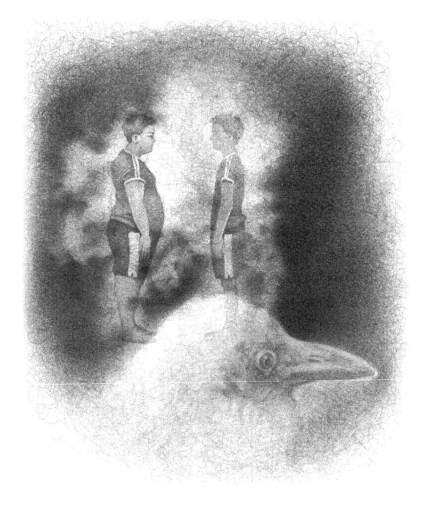

a flock of crows in her back yard. There were also bobwhites and doves, cooing to each other, and a woodpecker hammering on a nearby tree.

"The woods seems especially alive with wildlife this morning!" Thelma said to Jason as she opened the screen door and stepped onto the porch.

Just then another huge crow landed on the porch railing right in front of them. They were startled to see that it was a WHITE crow. Jason could see his reflection in the eyes of this giant bird. The crow's eyes mesmerized Jason and as he peered into them, he could see his future—like gazing at a crystal ball. Freaky!

Jason blinked and blinked again, hardly believing what he was seeing. In one eye, he saw himself as an adult—fit and lean, energetic and enthused about all the exciting adventures going on in his life. In the other eye, he saw himself as an overweight, lethargic . . . well . . . first-class loser who spent his time lying around watching TV reality shows and scarfing down processed food like hot wings, chips and soda.

Is this some kind of omen? Jason thought. The crow stared eerily back at him then flapped his wings and took off, luring Jason in the direction of the woods. So off he ran to explore and discover nature like he never had before. He vaulted over the railing and ran through the garden, where he grabbed a few ripe tomatoes and ate them like apples.

"Where you goin', boy?" Thelma yelled as Jason turned back and grinned at her.

"To the woods, where nothing can cage me," he said. "I've gotta get out of here!" As Jason headed for the park, he savored, as if for the first time, the sound of the wind in the trees, the murmur of insects and the singing of birds; it sounded sweeter than any tune he'd played on his portable music player, that's for sure.

And the scenery beat even his HDTV.

Thelma watched closely as Jason ran willy-nilly across the yard, the first time in ages since she'd seen him—or any young one—do that.

"Ah, finally!" she said aloud with a sigh. "Someone's running through my garden again!"

CHAPTER THREE

DOWN ON THE FARM

Sally stood in the center of her parent's garden, looking as fresh and sweet as the pink roses that surrounded her. Jason had always had a little crushy-crush on Sally since the first time he laid eyes on her in the neighbor's yard. Wow, had it really been five years since Sally's family moved into the farmhouse next to Thelma and William? Of course, Jason only got to see Sally when he was visiting his grandpa and grandma in Pennsylvania. When he was back home in upstate New York during the school year, he barely thought of Sally. But there she was, pretty as a picture, and Jason couldn't resist walking over to say hello.

"What's goin' on, Sally?" Jason said in greeting.

"Not too much, what's new with you, Jas?"

For some reason, Jason felt comfortable opening up to Sally about what happened to him the previous day with the white crow. Somehow, he knew she'd understand so he told her about the double visions he saw of his future self in the crow's eyes.

Sally's father knows all too well about the ravages of unhealthy eating on the body because he is a cardiologist at the local hospital. He's always preaching about the importance of good nutrition to Sally and her brothers. And Sally more than takes this to heart—and not just because her dad is a heart doctor. She's a competitive swimmer at her high school and wants to have the winning edge.

Jason shared his crow story as they walked together to a pond beyond Sally's yard.

"My grandma got me thinking about my eating habits and how often I'm inside on the computer but, I'll tell you what, that crow thing really tripped me out!" Jason commented.

Just as he said that, they stopped at the edge of the pond and gazed in.

"OMG! It's happening again!" Jason screeched as he saw an image of his fat future self reflecting back at him. "What the freak is going on???"

Sally's jaw dropped, too. "I think someone's trying to tell you something."

* * *

When Jason returned back to his grandparent's farmhouse, William was getting ready to go fishing. William didn't just fish for sport; he and Thelma ate everything he caught from the nearby freshwater lake. In fact, as an avid hunter and farmer, most of their diet was either home grown or hand caught. It began to dawn on Jason that it's no wonder his grandparents were fit as fiddles in their senior years. William was stronger than a team of oxen and he couldn't remember his grandma being sick even one day in her life. In fact, Old Lady Thelma didn't look old at all—she looked quite spry, almost youthful.

By contrast, Jason's mom, Mandy, and dad, Tom, seem "old" in their 50s. Both of them struggle with weight issues. Tom has high blood pressure and diabetes; Mandy has asthma and arthritic knees. Tom is a traveling salesman for a software company—part of the reason why Jason always has the latest technological gadgets—and he eats on the go, grabbing subs at the quickie-mart or a breakfast sandwich on his way to the office.

Mandy's job with a national insurance company is high-pressured, as well, leaving little time to prepare home cooked meals during the week. More often than she'd like to admit, Mandy tells Jason to grab a toaster pastry or microwavable breakfast sandwich on the way out the door; she's usually running late and wanting to beat rush hour traffic. When Jason gets off the school bus, what's waiting for him is a pantry full of processed, high-sugar snack foods that are easy to grab on the fly at the convenience store. Given no other choices, Jason binges on whatever's in the house because waiting until 7 o'clock or later to eat dinner with his parents seems like a long way off. As a result, Jason has grown pudgy.

Jason thought for a minute about how his mom was raised on the same farm where his grandparents still lived, and ate wholesome food growing up. Somehow, Mandy had gotten away from it when she left for college and started her career. It seems like by the time Jason came along, she had forgotten a lot of the good habits she learned as a farmer's daughter.

Empowered by the surreal image of himself in the pond as an overweight adult, Jason begins to think about making some changes, but he's not sure how yet.

"Hey Grandpa, want some company fishing?" Jason asks, running out to the barn where William is preparing his tackle box.

"Why, sure, Jas—grab that pole and can of night crawlers next to it."

That afternoon, inspired by the white crow encounter, Jason went fishing for some answers about what he could do to turn his life around, and possibly help his aging-before-their-time parents, as well. Grandpa was very wise and had a lot to say about the subject—and he's a great problem-solver. So, by the time they returned with their catch, William and Jason had hammered out a deal: Jason would return to Pennsylvania at the end of the school year, stay the entire summer, and William would pay him to help farm the fields. He'd teach him everything he knows about natural foods and working the land. What's more, Jason made a promise that each day, he would try to introduce something from the garden into his meals. It was going to be tough cause Jason also agreed to give up some of his favorite things for those three months: sodas, artificial sugary desserts and anything made with bleached, white flour.

Thelma agreed to set aside her summer evenings with her ladies' cross stitching circle to teach Jason all she knew about the ways of nature and the animal world, to which she had an obvious special connection. Thelma was very wise, too, and had oodles of experiences with fascinating stuff like plant spirits and animal totems. Jason had a sense that all of this tied in somehow with living a healthier life and having a prosperous future as an adult.

* * *

That spring, Jason began to collect books and other resources about leading-edge research on the possible adverse effects of the technological age—something that he was starting to become passionate about, as well. He loved technology but started to ponder how it could best be used for good reasons beyond just entertainment and convenience. The crow had a powerful message for Jason and he intended to fully explore it—even if he didn't quite know yet what it all meant.

By the time that the end of his high school sophomore year rolled around, Jason was totally psyched to experiment with changing his unhealthy habits for the better. Summer would be the perfect time to delve into all of this. And if he cleaned up his act and got fit, who knows? He might even win Sally's heart.

CHAPTER FOUR

THE SKINNY ON CHILDHOOD OBESITY

❝ For the first time in American history, children are expected to have a shorter life expectancy than their parents—and obesity is to blame."[1]

Jason read that statistic, looked down at the small gut hanging over his belt line then sat back in his chair. He couldn't get his mind around this. *Teenagers are supposed to be invincible, smarter than their parents,* he thought. *We're the generation that's going to change the world!* But this statistic did not compute in Jason's brain. *Die at a younger age than my parents? Sick!* He read on and learned that childhood obesity has become a national epidemic.

He went online and found studies that showed that childhood obesity has tripled since the 1980s, to the point that one in three children are overweight—and that percentage is still steadily rising. And the extra pounds are taking a toll on kids' health. It's causing them to have sleep apnea, social and psychological problems such as poor self-esteem, as well as bone and joint problems. According to the Centers for Disease Control, 70 percent of overweight children between the ages of five and 17 already have at least one risk factor for heart disease, including elevated blood cholesterol, blood pressure or increased insulin levels; these

---

1 Alliance for a Healthier Generation, www.healthiergeneration.org

are exactly the factors that lead to hypertension, diabetes, stroke, several types of cancer and osteoarthritis.[2]

Another study that Jason came across showed that increasing numbers of kids need prescription drugs to reduce their odds of heart disease—meds that used to be used almost exclusively by adults to control high blood pressure and diabetes. Startlingly, the biggest increase in the use of these meds is occurring in the youngest group studied: 6 to 11 year olds. Then Jason came across other research that found that one in five American four-year-olds—yes, preschoolers—is obese. If left untreated, the studies noted, kids' fast-food diets, lack of exercise and growing weight problems could lead to full blown heart disease, high blood pressure, cancers and joint diseases by age 30.

Could the news get much worse? Well, Jason also tracked down data online that revealed that people who are overweight or obese in young adulthood (and middle-age) are at elevated risk of being disabled in their later years. The longer a person has been overweight, the greater their risk of mobility limitations—and injury. The bones and muscles of obese children are more vulnerable because of increased body mass and force, making them more likely to twist or roll on an extremity and cause injury. Is this the future that Jason had to look forward to . . . or, dread?

"Man, that would suck," he said aloud to himself.

It all made Jason wonder how he fit into the definition of obesity, so he delved further into his research. He learned that a child is considered to be obese if their body-mass index, a height-weight ratio, was in the 95th percentile or higher based on government BMI growth charts. Basically, a boy is obese if his body weight is more than 25 percent fat; a girl, more than 32 percent. Said another way, if a child's weight is 20 percent or more in

---

2 Centers for Disease Control, www.cdc.gov

excess of the expected weight for a given height, he is considered to be mildly obese. If his weight is 30 percent or more above the desirable body weight, he is considered to be severely obese.

Jason was curious about his own BMI and so he researched a way to calculate it. While the BMI percentile charts that he found online were a good way for Jason to familiarize himself with these tools, he also learned that calculating this at home with a scale and tape measure is not an accurate assessment; he would have to have his measurements taken at his pediatrician's office or during his school physical, because evidently even small measuring mistakes can result in big errors in BMI calculations. Still, Jason used the charts to get a general idea of where he stood health-wise.

"By government standards, I'm considered mildly obese," Jason said to his parents the following weekend when he was able to finally get them to take time out of their hectic schedules and talk with him about his newfound obsession.

"Oh, you are *not!*" Mandy said in reaction. "You just still have a little baby fat, dear. You'll grow out if it."

"Denial is a dangerous thing, Mom, a dangerous thing." Jason said, only half joking.

"Denial? Denial of what?"

"Mom, did you know that the most valuable weapon a kid has in the battle against childhood obesity is parents who model self-control and good choices with their own eating habits?"

"Huh? Jas! What are you saying to me?"

"I'm just sayin'. . . denial is a dangerous thing."

"Maybe you have a point, son," Tom chimed in. "I know I don't have the healthiest eating habits, and it's not good—for me or for you guys."

"So what would you like me to do?" Mandy said, a bit testy.

"I have a suggestion," Jason added. "Let's just agree to do one thing, just one small step to get us headed back in the right direction—cause I'm not going to outgrow this 'baby fat' and, uh, well, you guys aren't getting any younger."

"Oh, thanks a lot, Jas," Mandy said. "What's your big idea?"

* * *

Jason learned that Americans today drink about twice as many calories as they did in the previous generation. Sugar-sweetened beverages are a major downfall among American dieters. This equates roughly to 235 to 450 per day, or nearly an extra half-pound to a pound of fat gain in a week! So why not just drink diet soda? Because that doesn't solve the problem, Jason learned. Emerging research suggests that consuming sugary-tasting beverages—even if they're artificially sweetened—can lead to a hankering for sweetness overall—including sweeter (and more caloric) cereal, bread, dessert, everything. Diet soda is 100 percent nutrition-free and there are concerns about aspartame, which is a whopping 180 times sweeter than sugar. Some animal research has linked its consumption in high quantities to brain tumors and lymphoma in rodents. Yea, the FDA says the sweetener is safe, but even Jason has to admit he's had some of the reported side effects from drinking too much of it: dizziness, mood swings, headaches, diarrhea and intestinal discomfort.

"Yea, it should be called die-it soda," Jason quipped to his parents that day.

"That decides it then," Tom responded. "We're officially off soda."

"Cool. If we do nothing else between now and the beginning of summer, this will be it. Deal?"

"Deal," Tom agreed. Mandy shrugged her approval.

Jason decided to instead drink the most natural thing available: water. By the time June rolled around, making just than one change, Jason and his parents dropped a collective 20 pounds and felt much better physically, too. But Jason was just getting started. *How fabulous could I feel by the end of summer,* he wondered?

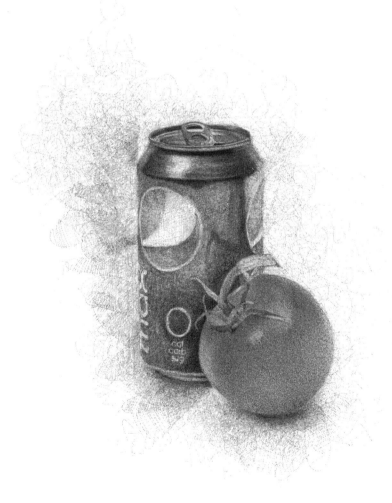

CHAPTER FIVE

WHO'S YOUR MAMA? MOTHER EARTH

"Green Acres is the place to be!" William sang, quoting an old sitcom tune that was televised long before Jason was a glint in his mother's eye. "I know it sounds backwards but more folks are wising up to their agricultural roots," he suggested to Jason as they sat on the front porch swing and sipped fresh-squeezed lemonade in the morning sun.

"What do you mean, Grandpa?"

"I'm not making this up. I just read a feature in a major national daily newspaper about the trend of families fleeing the rat race and adopting a more self-reliant lifestyle. If these past few years have shown our country anything, it's that we can't count on a stable economy; we can only count on ourselves. Ha, funny that it's taken a recession to inspire families and young single folks to head back to the country. Yep, buying a nice piece of land. Growing your own food. Raising your own chickens and pigs. That's what's real, boy. And don't forget it. People are catching on. In fact, the rural population of folks ages 55 to 85 is due to increase by 30 percent by the year 2020."

"But Grandpa, nobody wants to go back to the old days before technology," Jason said.

"Technology can be a blessing or a curse."

"What d'ya mean?"

"We have all these gadgets, appliances and machines that are sleek microprocessor-controlled wonders but what happens when the power goes out or the satellite signal gets interrupted? Everything goes mute and motionless. We become powerless."

"Hmmm...Good point. Guess I never thought about Big Grid failure!"

"Yea, I've been thinking a lot about this, especially as it relates to our country's food supply. Technology can advance or it can destroy. Over the years, I've seen many farms destroyed by modern farming practices that kill native plant cover, deplete the topsoil, strip it of nutrients, and further degrade it by the use of pesticides and chemical fertilizers."

"Well, why can't we combine the best of modern technology with old-fashioned self-reliance to come up with a better way to live?"

"Yea, the good news is that advances in biointensive farming offer sustainable alternatives to chemical-intensive farming. This would actually increase productivity while replenishing the soil. Unfortunately, agribusiness continues to deplete the topsoil and pollute the environment. I see it every day. We're not taking care of Mother Earth."

"It sounds like a huge problem. What can anyone do?"

"Support organic farmers and other planet-friendly practices. This change has to be consumer led. We've forgotten that we each have power—the power of our pocket books."

All of this intrigued Jason and spurred him to look even further into natural eating—not just for his own health but the health of the planet and everyone on it. In his World Cultures class that school year, he had studied about ancient civilizations and learned that for at least 100,000 generations, tribal cultures have existed across the planet, living in sustainable harmony with

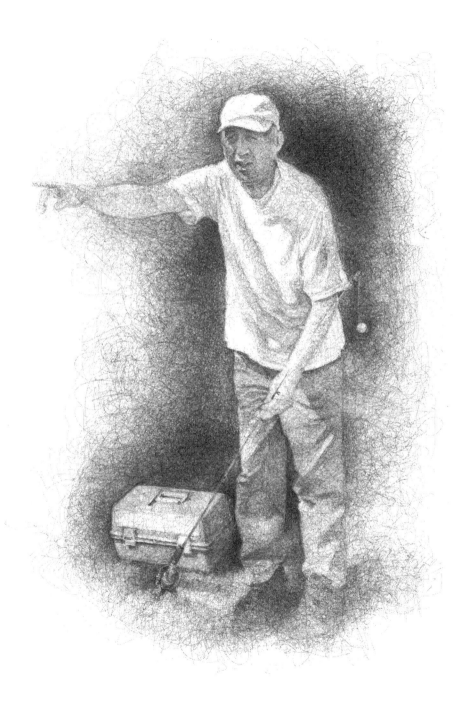

nature. They lived on fruits, vegetables and lean meats—the foods varied with the seasons and climate, and all of it was obtained from local sources. And he learned that before the advent of penicillin and other modern medicine, archaeological records indicate that hunter-gatherers averaged five to six inches taller, had more teeth left at the time of their death and lived longer than even agricultural people. While 500 generations have depended on agriculture, only 10 generations have lived since the onset of the industrial age, and only two have grown up with highly processed fast foods. What does this all mean? To Jason, it all definitely seemed to point back to the problem of obesity and that daunting statistic that his generation would have a shorter life expectancy than the previous one.

"Well, enough thinkin' for one day . . . let's get workin'," William said, getting up off the swing and heading towards the barn. "Those cows need milkin'. And you're in charge of the milk cows for the entire summer!" he reminded Jason.

Jason followed behind him, grabbed a pail and stool, and got started with the morning chores—all the while, pondering the big picture of humankind and how we got to this era where we're smart enough to invent microprocessors that give us the world in the palm of our hands, but blind enough to be mass producing food that is slowly killing us.

CHAPTER SIX

THELMA TELLS ALL

"Every animal has a powerful spirit that communicates messages to us," Thelma said as she and Jason strolled through the woods one early Sunday morning. "Ah! We can learn so much from creatures and critters and the natural world—it's like having everything we need to know about the secret to life all around us—it's just a matter of noticing it."

"Um, I couldn't help but notice that albino crow last year, and now I'm seeing crows all the time, even in the school parking lot."

"Then the crow is probably your totem right now."

"My what?"

"Your animal totem, or 'power animal.' When a certain wild creature comes into your life repeatedly, you know it's time to pay attention to its lessons. Your power animal chooses you—not the other way around—so now you need to read about crow medicine and honor its wisdom."

"So what does it mean that I have crows around me, Grandma?"

"I think the crow is the smartest of all birds. It can outwit most other birds, animals and even humans. Crows have great intelligence and can adapt easily to their environment."

"So the crow is telling me to be smart and adaptable?"

"Yes, but actually, crow medicine reminds us that the secret magic of creation is calling us. Its caw is a reminder that creation and the natural world are cawing out to us every day. Jason dear, I think you are being summoned to reconnect with nature!"

"Cool. I definitely feel that. I mean, I'm living here for the summer and farming with you and Grandpa. It's something I hadn't considered doing until now, even though you two invite me to stay every year. I guess crows DO have some special magic!"

"You're lucky, Jason, cause nowadays, the average person doesn't understand this important connection, especially young ones. They live in cloistered environments in cities and carefully manicured suburbs with artificial lights and central heating—away from the wild and the truly natural world. Being in nature loosens up our 'natural' gifts of creativity, imagination and adaptability, and lets us run free with them—however we choose to do that. It saddens me that a lot of kids your age have lost that connection."

"Yea, I would say most of my friends don't even notice things around them like birds and wild animals. And if they don't have a chance to interact with them, they can't 'get the message,' right?"

"And it's not just animals—everything in nature speaks to us. Listen," Thelma said, motioning for Jason to be quiet and still. They stood, silent, in their tracks for several minutes. "Oh yes, the trees and plants and shrubs and creatures are silently crying."

"You can *hear* that?"

"Uh huh. They're whispering, 'Where are all the children? They used to play in the woods, climb our trees, swim in our ponds and rivers'!"

"Come on, Grandma, the trees aren't really saying that!"

"Really? Well, maybe by the end of summer, you'll be able

to hear what I hear when I walk through the woods."

* * *

As they came upon a clearing, Thelma spread a blanket for her and Jason to sit on. While they relaxed and enjoyed the sunshine, Thelma enlightened Jason about how animals in the wild use their instincts and creativity to adapt and live healthily in their environment.

"When they're sick, they self-medicate by eating certain roots, bark, clay and leaves, and drinking water," she explained. "They use grasses and rough leaves as scours and emetics. You see, there's such a thing as plant medicine, too. Plants can heal. For instance, one plant that even dogs commonly eat is goldenrod, which is a natural anti-inflammatory and has antiseptic properties. Animals know to avoid certain poisonous plants, predators and poor food choices—they know what they need to do to stay alive."

Thelma went on to explain that animals raised in captivity, unable to range freely over their natural habitat, don't fare as well and have shorter life spans. "Did you know that nearly half of zoo gorillas die of cardiovascular disease, and many are infertile or suffer eating disorders?" she asked. "Captive elephants develop foot problems and arthritis, and often lack the urge to mate. Captive giraffes suffer from excessive hoof growth."

"Because of the food they're given?" Jason asked.

"Yes, diet accounts for much of the ill health of animals in zoos. Captive woolly monkeys commonly die of kidney and liver failure caused by an inadequate diet. Many carnivores and primates suffer obesity and persistent diarrhea, along with tooth and urinary problems. Captive reptiles get rickets and osteoporosis. Often the animals stop eating altogether and have to be force-fed. But it's not just their diet that's the problem, it's also that captive animals don't get the appropriate amount of natural sunlight and exercise."

"What does a lack of sunlight cause?"

"Everything from bone deformities to captive primates cannibalizing their litters."

"What? They eat their babies?"

"Uh huh. Maybe it's instinctual cause they know their offspring will not be healthy or even able to survive. So you're getting my drift here, right Jas? People are the same way: being in an artificial environment and ingesting unnatural food can make anyone a little crazy. That's why having a connection to nature and its bounty is so important. Also, think about this: when your buddies are being held captive by their TVs and computers and other electronics, they're not getting adequate exercise, either."

"Yea, that's been my problem. I'm a TV junkie."

"The California naturalist Ian McMillan says that the cult of wilderness is not a luxury, it's a necessity for our own protection and for the preservation of our mental health! In captive animals, the lack of social interaction leads to boredom, psychological disturbances and even violence and self-abuse."

"Okay now you're really describing my buddies, Grandma!"

"Ah, then I need to send a shaman over to visit them and help them see their unhealthy ways."

"A what?"

"A shaman is a person who serves as a messenger between the natural and spirit worlds. They are natural healers and they can unlock the spirits inside of you. Some shamans do this by using animal and plant medicine. They believe that each organ in our body has a spirit, and the only way to unlock it is to be in nature. A shaman could inspire your friends to get away from their electronic cages and go outside."

"Hmmm.... Why do my buddies need a shaman, Grandma, when I can just send YOU to their homes!" Jason quipped.

"Better yet," she said, "Let's have our crow friend send them a message . . . "

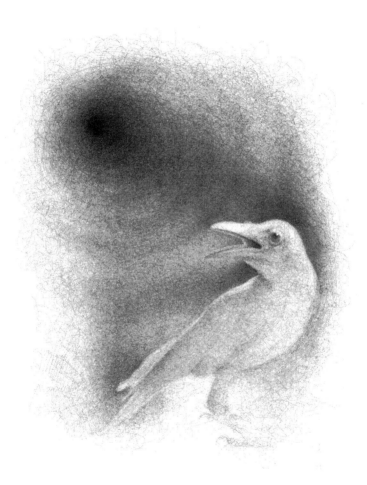

CHAPTER SEVEN

WILLIAM'S HARVEST OF KNOWLEDGE

Plant medicine. Food as medicine. Hmmm . . . Jason rolled this over in his mind. It's certainly a far cry from the way he'd always viewed food. Eating was something that he did out of hunger, obviously, but also out of habit. Eating was often for entertainment and as long as his belly was full, he didn't care too much how it got that way. He definitely didn't think of food as fuel, as energy, as something that could heal him . . . or worse yet, harm him if he wasn't eating the proper stuff.

To the contrary, how much fast food Jason and his friends could consume was a matter of pride, of teenage intestinal fortitude. Now Thelma had him thinking about how "alive" plants are versus how "dead" a greasy burger is. Come to think of it, now that he'd sworn off junk food and sugary "energy drinks" for the summer and replaced them with meals that mostly consisted of freshly grown fruits and vegetables from the farm, Jason had to admit that HE felt more alive, too. He was quickly getting used to picking snap peas from the vine and eating them right on the spot. The scent of fresh basil and ripe Big Boy tomatoes in Thelma's kitchen garden was mildly intoxicating—he couldn't get enough whiffs as he walked by them. And the potatoes that William sliced up in the oven with a bit of herbs and olive oil were better than any French fries he'd ever eaten. His meals were fresh and vibrant

. . . what a concept! By contrast, how many miles and how many days did the meat in those fast-food burgers have to travel before they came off the assembly line?

"It's all a racket," Jason protested to his mom on the phone that morning. "Did you ever notice, Mom, how many commercials that air during the Saturday morning kids shows are for foods that are high in fat, grease, salt and sugar?"

"Uh, probably as many commercials as there are for medications during the adult prime time programming," Mandy joked.

"I just read somewhere that one out of every three toys given to a child in the United States each year is from a fast-food restaurant. What's that tell you?"

"Uh, uh . . ." Mandy didn't know how to answer because she was guilty of placating her son with a plastic contraption of the latest animated movie character—which happened to come with chicken nuggets and fries—and calling it "dinner" at least one night every week when Jason was in grade school.

"Geesh, you sound like the neighborhood anti-junk food evangelist these days, Jas."

"Well, Grandma and I watched the movie *Super Size Me* last week and . . ."

"Wait . . . Grandma actually let you watch TV?"

"Well just the DVD of the movie . . . anyway, the main guy in the movie, Morgan Spurlock, ate nothing but fast food for an entire month. He looked and felt like crap at the end of his experiment and the doctors told him that his liver had already begun to malfunction—after only one month!"

"Ugh."

"And Grandpa has me reading a book called *Chew On This: Everything You Don't Want to Know About Fast Food*. It mentions that people who live in Okinawa off the coast of Japan have the healthiest diet in the world—mostly fish, fruits, vegetables and soy protein, and small amounts of meat. People in Okinawa have always lived longer than just about anyone anywhere else in the world, well over 100 years old. Then in the 1970s after the first fast-food restaurant opened and the presence of U.S. military bases encouraged people there to adopt an American diet, everything changed. Now Okinawa has the highest obesity rate in Japan. Their life expectancy is falling. And many of the elders there who never learned to like fast food and still eat the island's traditional foods will probably outlive their children."

While Jason was away for the summer, Mandy and Tom made a commitment to themselves to try and eat healthier, too. It had become an imperative since Mandy's doctor warned her that given the track she was on, she would need to begin taking daily medication for high blood pressure and cholesterol in a few years. The extra weight was also causing her to have pain in her knees and ankles. She and Tom followed Jason's simple advice to grocery shop as if they were choosing items from Grandpa's garden—mostly in-season fruits and vegetables with a "side" of protein like lean meat or fish. Jason also gave his parents a couple of good resources for reading food labels so they could literally see what they were eating.

"Better yet," he told his mom and dad, "eat mostly food that doesn't need a label at all. I mean, you look at a banana and you know what's in it . . . a banana!"

* * *

Sally couldn't believe her eyes. Jason seemed to have transformed from a boy to a young man since she last saw him the previous summer. For some reason, he looked really cute to her now. Was it that his hair was longer and blonde-streaked from the sun? The killer tan he had going on looked good, too, and she knew it wasn't because he'd been lounging by the pool—she had seen Jason in the fields with his grandfather, plowing and planting rows of crops.

"Hey there, you!" Jason shouted as he jogged over to Sally's yard.

Feeling suddenly shy, she glanced at Jason's body then looked away.

"What's up, Sally?"

"Uh, not much. It's really good to see you. You look, I don't know, different."

"Yea?"

Sally couldn't help but notice that Jason was slimmer, more toned. He'd grown a few inches, too, but it was more than that. He seemed more confident, really energized and, well, he had kind of a glow about him, like an aura of light or something.

"Yea. You look great."

"Uh, you want to go berry picking later, like after dinner?"

"Sure. Where?

"It's just beyond the corn field. My grandma has a huge patch of raspberries and blueberries. Some of the raspberries should be ripe by now. Six thirty okay?"

"Yea."

"Cool."

"Okay, well, I need to go. My swim team has practice in an hour. We have a meet next month. It's a pretty big deal. I'm sort of excited about it."

"Wow, that's awesome, Sally. Maybe I can come and watch?"

"Sure, I'd like that."

"Okay."

"Cool, well, have fun at practice. I'll see you at six thirty."

"Thanks. Later."

Jason turned and walked on air back towards the farm and did a one-arm leap over the split rail fence. Nothing could quite make Jason's day like a smile from Sally. And this time, for the first time, he felt her smile all the way into his heart.

CHAPTER EIGHT

JASON'S JUNIOR YEAR CAMPAIGN

By the time Jason's junior year began, he had educated himself on various dietary guidelines, including the USDA's MyPyramid and the New Four Food Groups (proposed in 1991 by the Physicians' Committee for Responsible Medicine). Not only was Jason eating mostly grains, fruits, vegetables and legumes, he had weaned himself off processed, high-calorie foods and snacks, as well as the need to always be in front of some form of an electronic device. Okay, sure, he had his cell phone on him at all times, texting friends day and night. But he hadn't played one video game since he stepped foot on the farm at the beginning of summer, and because he was busy with daily chores and doing things outdoors, he found himself firing up his laptop and turning on the TV less and less. In fact, when he did go online, it was for a productive reason: to search the Internet for information related to his newfound "human experiment."

Yes, Jason had taken himself on as a sort of science project. How good could he feel by eating only fresh, nourishing foods? How fit could he get by doing natural manual labor like farming and building tree huts and repairing the wood siding on the horse barn, supplemented by a workout routine (which he also researched online)? He discovered favorite websites that even had recipes for easy-to-make meals and "real" energy drinks like smoothies made from fresh fruits.

Admittedly, the New Four Food Groups was a departure from the diet that Jason was raised on, but it was very close to the kind that his grandparents lived every day. It's basically:

Fruit: 3 or more servings a day

Legumes (or, beans, peas, lentils, etc.):

    2 or more servings a day

Whole grains: 5 or more servings a day

Vegetables: 4 or more servings a day

The diet is purposely devoid of two food groups: meat and dairy. At first, Jason found this to be challenging so he initially decided to limit his intake of items in these two food groups instead of cutting them out completely. But then he read something that caused him to flip his perspective about this: he came across the recipes in a groundbreaking book by Neal Barnard, MD called *Food for Life: How the New Four Food Groups Can Save Your Life.* He found it surprisingly easy to concoct all kinds of meals that were inexpensive and remarkably delicious—things like whole-wheat pancakes, berry cobbler, vegetable stew, tamale pie, buckwheat pasta and banana cake. He discovered through Dr. Barnard's book that it's simple to replace unhealthy stuff like refined sugar, oils and animal fat with more wholesome alternatives like almond and rice milk, unsweetened fruit preserves, vegetable broth, and even two meat substitutes—"seitan," which is made from wheat and "tempah," made from soybeans—that could be used to whip up all kinds of typically meat-based meals. With so many options and alternatives, Jason didn't feel that he needed meat or dairy to have a satisfying, nutritious diet.

* * *

When Jason walked into class on the first day of the new school year, his friends couldn't believe his transformation. They all wanted to know how he got so fit, and he was happy to share what he'd learned. His teachers were impressed, too, and by the end of the first semester, his physical fitness teacher asked him to help stage an assembly that the school was hosting for the freshmen and sophomore classes on healthy lifestyle habits. Jason created a presentation and called it "Energy Leaks: How Fake Food and Electronic Devices Insidiously Ravage Our Health Until We Die"—a pretty intense title but, hey, teenagers live on drama.

"Did you know that the grease from French fries takes three months to exit your body?" he asked his audience during the assembly. "Yea, if you've eaten at a fast-food establishment anytime since the first day of school, those French fries are still in your gut right now, all fermented and putrid. Gross, huh?

"Even 'normal' foods like milk and chicken are now tainted because industrialized food producers inject steroids and growth hormones into their live farm animals, which are carried down the food chain when we consume this stuff. There's a lot you don't know if you're not keeping up with this stuff—that's how I 'spent my summer vacation' and it's amazing what I learned about what's going on behind the isles of our nation's grocery stores.

"Like the way food is packaged and labeled . . . When you're pouring your cereal in the morning before the bus comes, I'm sure you're not measuring a half-cup as your serving size, as the food manufacturers recommend. You're probably dumping twice or three times the amount listed on the label—which means you have to double or triple the amount of sugar, fat, carbs, sodium, calories and everything else listed on the label."

Jason asked for a show of hands to see how many classmates feel that they often need a sugary drink fix like a mega-calorie energy drink or gourmet coffee beverage. Not surprisingly, nearly everyone raised their hands.

"I'm not saying you can't have a large mocha frappe every once in a while," he cautioned, "just keep in mind that those drinks contain about 500 calories and 24 grams of fat—which is more fat and sugar than a huge hunk of strawberry cheesecake. Skip the coffee drink and go back to eating a healthy breakfast like fresh fruit with oatmeal or a wheat English muffin with peanut butter."

* * *

The second half of Jason's presentation made the connection between unhealthy eating and how technology is making kids lazy.

"Computers and cell phones and computer games and HDTV and all that stuff is cool," he went on to tell his young audience. "What's NOT cool is when you're attached to these 'high-speed pipes' all the time. Think about it: our homes have become entertainment hubs but because we don't have to go anywhere to get any of this stuff, they're more like caves. We're staring at computers and TV screens instead of socializing. We're sitting on the couch instead of out running around and moving our bodies. And how many of you are usually eating some kind of processed food while you're loafing on the couch?" Jason asked for a show of hands again. Mostly everyone responded.

"Exactly. All it's doing is leading you straight down the path to diabetes, heart disease, high blood pressure and other health conditions—and these things are all preventable. Even the First Lady of the United States agrees with me," Jason added, explaining that the White House, led by Michelle Obama, instituted a sweeping campaign called "Let's Move" to revamp the way American children eat and play—reshaping school lunches, playgrounds and even medical checkups—with the goal of eliminating childhood obesity within a generation.

"Mrs. Obama was right when she said, 'The truth is, our kids didn't choose to make food products with tons of fat and sugar and super-size portions, and then to have those foods marketed to them wherever they turn'."

Jason wrapped up his presentation with a warning and a call to action. "I'm here to tell you that young adults like you and me are being force-fed a steady stream of brain-scrubbing messages about food when we watch TV. It's true: food manufacturers are using shameless and seductive marketing tactics to trap us into buying kid-targeted junk food that is having a huge negative impact on our food preferences and eating habits. It's time to protest! How do we protest? By not buying this type of food!"

Jason went on to explain that the Federal Trade Commission made a valiant effort back in the 1970s (the Dark Ages) to regulate advertisements for other products that are hazardous to our health. A precedent was set with the ban of TV ads for cigarettes and liquor but the FTC encountered a congressional roadblock that proved to be insurmountable. Since then the number of child-targeted food commercials has skyrocketed and so have the number of overweight children.

"As a result, all you need to know, guys, is this: the more TV you watch, the more fat and calories your diets will contain and the more likely you are to become overweight. So what's the word, dudes? Get off the freakin' couch and get busy doing something outdoors! Need some ideas? Here's something to get you started . . . I need your support!"

With that, Jason handed out papers for each student to help him going door-to-door in his community to petition for healthier lunches and healthy snacks in the vending machines at his school. A small crowd of students came to the front of the auditorium to express their interest in helping out. Jason had hoped that everyone would get involved but he knew this was a grassroots effort. And that's how the groundswell starts: one person at a time.

* * *

Back at home, Jason began teaching his parents what he'd learned the previous summer on grandpa's farm and they were game to make changes. He and his parents were now sitting down more often for family meals and eating less on the fly. Jason pitched in to help prepare dinner before his parents arrived home from work, and both Mandy and Tom made it a point to leave the office by 5 p.m. at least one night each week—even going in earlier if necessary to keep their promise to Jason.

The family kept the TV off while having dinner and didn't snack past 9 p.m. unless it was a special occasion. Mandy had taken to drinking green tea in the morning instead of coffee and sodas, and Tom made sure he drank six to eight glasses of water each day while at work. Jason and his mom were now taking walks after dinner when possible—good bonding time for the two of them—and Tom finally took his friends up on their offer to join their pick-up basketball games two evenings a week at the local gymnasium.

Jason also informed Mandy and Tom about the research he'd done on portion control. He'd read that U.S. portion sizes are at an all time high and these larger portions encourage overeating by as much as 56 percent. The super-sizing of foods and beverages in U.S. restaurants and fast food chains is at least partially to blame for the upsizing of Americans, who typically eat at least three meals a week away from home. In a survey conducted by the American Institute for Cancer Research, one-third of Americans polled said that the more they're served, the more they tend to eat. In the same survey, 70 percent of American adults said that when they're dining out, they almost always polish off everything on their plates.

And eating too many calories at one meal doesn't necessarily lead to settling for fewer calories at the next one, as Jason could personally attest. Of course, the amount of food served at home is easier to control. To avoid overeating, Jason learned, always eat from plates and bowls, not directly from the box or bag. So Jason suggested that his parents serve meals on smaller dishes, which is what they did. It was too simple of an experiment to not try, and it ended up working because no one missed the extra food that wasn't on their plates.

All the while that Jason was helping his parents relearn healthy eating habits, he was keeping copious notes about every-thing they were doing and tracking everyone's progress, including his own. His family had collectively lost another 35 pounds that year. But more than that, they each felt more physically and men-tally energized. Even better than that, eating more meals together and sharing in the preparation of those meals was somehow bring-ing them closer together as a family. It was a really good thing, and Jason wanted that to continue—especially since he knew that in one more year, he'd be graduated and off to college.

CHAPTER NINE

THE CROW'S RETURN

At the end of Jason's junior year, he returned to his grandparent's farm . . . and to Sally, who wasn't quite "his girl" yet but he was working on it. That summer, one of his goals was to devise an aggressively healthy eating plan for Sally to follow during her upcoming competitive swimming season. A big scholarship to a state university was on the line for Sally and she had every intention of besting her personal best that year so that she could nail the scholarship—so she asked Jason for his help with nutrition. He was happy to oblige, going so far as to cook dinner a couple of times that summer for Sally and her parents. Even "doctor dad" was impressed, and Jason was certainly making a good impression on Sally, too.

By now, Jason had become a young shaman in his own right. Although he had so much to learn and understand about the biology and chemistry of good nutrition, he was quickly becoming a "natural" at farming and the "business" of food. In fact, he was seriously considering studying agriculture at a four-year university after graduation this coming year. But first, he had one more summer under grandpa's tutelage and he wanted to plant his own crops for sale at harvest time that August—which is exactly what he did. The extra money he earned came in handy and he made some good contacts at the local farmer's markets with other folks who lived an agrarian lifestyle.

* * *

It's a no-brainer that by the time Jason had to pick a subject for his senior project, he decided to take everything he'd learned on his own—along with all the information he'd tracked at home the previous year and the plan he'd devised for Sally—and put it into a formalized program for anyone to follow. He titled part of his plan "Jason's 10 Interactive Exercises to Whip Kids into Shape" and staged a "New Four Food Groups cook-off" as part of his project during the spring of his senior year. What a night it was! Students, teachers, parents and a few dignitaries from the community (the mayor included!) came together at a neighborhood restaurant to invent and prepare recipes ala Food Network's *Top Chef* and *Hell's Kitchen*. Even more people paid to come and taste the recipes. Jason earmarked the evening's proceeds to benefit a farmer's relief fund based in Pennsylvania, near his grandparent's farm. A good time was had by everyone and it was all for a good cause.

* * *

Before long, Jason was donning his cap and gown for high school graduation. On the evening of commencements, as the high school principal presented Jason's diploma and shook his hand, a certain magic filled the air. It had stormed earlier that afternoon and now the ragged, wistful rain clouds had given way to rays of light, causing an evanescent glow to descend upon the football stadium where the ceremony was being held. Jason graciously accepted his diploma and started to walk back to his seat. Just then, his eyes fixated on an arc of color emanating from one of the clouds . . . a rainbow so vivid that a chill ran up Jason's spine. Looking into the crowd, he spotted some familiar faces. Tom clapped hard and gave Jas a proud, approving smile. Mandy, who looked trimmer and younger than she had in years, swiped tears of joy from her face. And there was sweetie pie Sally, who traveled all the way from Pennsylvania with Thelma and William for Jason's big day. All five of them were precious to Jason and he wanted them to stay healthy and well for a very, very long time. He felt more passionate than ever about this.

As Jason found his way back to his seat, he felt profoundly grateful for the opportunity he'd been given during the past few years to turn his own life and health around, and "return to the natural world." Looking to the future, he was even more grateful that he could see a career path ahead of him using technology to improve the health of the planet and the way we grow food. Yes, Jason had decided to study agricultural science in college.

These types of scientists study farm crops and animals and develop ways to improve crop yield, control pests and weeds more safely and effectively, and conserve soil and water. They research methods of converting raw agricultural commodities into attractive and healthy food products for consumers. Jason could see himself working in the food processing industry, at a university or even with the federal government to create and improve food products. This field combined his love of biology, chemistry, physics, engineering and biotechnology. One day, he might develop a better way to preserve, process, package, store or deliver food. He might work as a researcher to discover new food sources, or ways to remove harmful additives from food or halt the spread of an insect-borne disease. Maybe he'll end up working as a food scientist who inspects food processing areas to ensure that sanitation, safety, quality and waste management standards are met.

Jason's ultimate dream is to become a plant scientist (ah, Thelma would be so happy!) to help food producers feed a growing population with close-to-the-ground foods and conserve natural resources. He would love to work directly with farmers just like William and other landowners about the best use of land and plants to avoid or correct problems such as soil erosion or pest migration.

Jason continued to ponder all of these career possibilities as he visited Thelma and William on the farm one last time before heading out west for college.

"We're proud of you, boy," William said, giving Jason a hearty slap on the back for good measure.

"Oh yes, dear, you've done good," Thelma chimed in. "Now, keep doin' it! Use the most of the talent God gave you and the good health that you've given yourself!"

Jason could hardly believe how much he'd grown up and changed in the past few years. At the same time, he found great comfort in the constancy of his grandparent's farm and how some things will always remain: the cackle of the roosters calling on the dawn, the smack of cow peat hitting his nostrils, the creak of the barn doors opening and the sensation of running willy nilly through Thelma's garden. Suddenly, he had an urge to do this one last time, while he could, just because . . . and right on cue in the nearby woods, up in the trees, egging him on . . . was a crow, caw-caw-cawing, as if to say, "Return to me, Return to me..."

PART II:

JASON'S 10 INTERACTIVE EXERCISES FOR WHIPPING KIDS INTO SHAPE

The following activities—which Jason created out of the goodness of his heart and smartness of his brain for the rest of his high school class (and for a passing grade)—can be used by children and adults alike. They will enhance communication skills and help participants explore the world of food and the wonder of nature. Each one will serve to help you make healthier life choices.

1. Explore Your Natural Surroundings

Research suggests that being in nature reduces stress in our daily lives, regardless of our age. Many of us have forgotten what it's like to be in nature. This exercise reminds us of its glory and reconnects us with the outside world. Exploring your surroundings can be a natural stepping stone into a healthier lifestyle.

◎ TIME

20 minutes per day

◎ MATERIALS

Place to walk or sit outside
Pen or pencil
Small pocket notebook
Watch or timer

◎ DIRECTIONS

1. Take a 15-minute walk.
2. Observe the sights (weather, colors, plants, animals), sounds and smells experienced while you walk.
3. Return from your walk and for five minutes, write in your notebook a list of words that describe your experience.

◎ TECHNOLOGY ALTERNATE

1. Create an online diary or blog to record your experiences.

Note to parents or staff utilizing this exercise. Once we lose touch with the benefits of wide-open spaces, a reintroduction is necessary in order for our senses to return to their natural ability to balance stress. Provide writing paper with this exercise so that participants can log the sensations of smell, sight, touch, hearing and feeling while walking or sitting quietly in a nature. As the parent or staff member, engage in this exercise with your participants so they understand what you are asking them to experience. One requirement for this exercise could be to have the person to sit or walk in his own space. For safety, walking can be done in pairs with limited interaction.

2. Get to Know Fruits and Vegetables . . . and Whole Grains and Pastas

There are such fabulous fruits, vegetables, whole grains and pastas available on the market today—get to know them! Fruits and vegetables, as well as whole grains and pastas, provide essential nutrients and fiber for healthy eating. Combining new fruits, vegetables and pastas can spark new food choices and add an element of surprise in encouraging healthy food choices.

◎ TIME

30 minutes per fruit or vegetable
(repeat with whole grains and pastas)

◎ MATERIALS

A fruit or vegetable
Utensils to peel or cut the fruit or vegetable
Serving plates, bowls and utensils
Pen and paper

◎ DIRECTIONS

1. Take a trip to the local farmer's market or grocery store.
2. Select a fruit or vegetable that is new to you.
3. Return home and set a three-minute timer.
4. Write down the characteristics of that fruit or vegetable, it's color, texture and size.
5. Peel or cut the fruit or vegetable.
6. Taste it, really taste it.
7. Write down words that come to you while eating the fruit or vegetable.
8. Write a short rap song about your selected fruit or vegetable.
9. Share your song with others.

◎ TECHNOLOGY ALTERNATE

1. Select fruits and vegetables that are new to you.
2. Search the Internet for pictures of these fruits and vegetables.
3. Create an online album of these pictures.
4. Share the album with others.

Note to parents or staff utilizing this exercise. An alternative to this exercise would be having a fruit-tasting contest in which participants talk about their fruit—the texture, taste, color, etc.—and suggest it as an alternative to candy. Or have a contest using dark chocolate versus milk chocolate candy with the idea that if you're going to go for something sweet, choose something (like dark chocolate) that has some nutritional value.

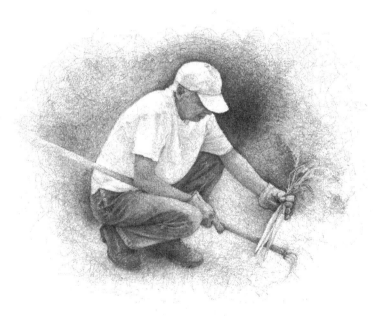

3. Measure Your Body Mass Index (BMI)

This can be a real eye-opener for both children and adults! BMI is an internationally used measurement of proper weight and obesity developed by Belgium statistician Adolphe Quetelet. Only two measurements are needed to determine your BMI: weight and height.

Adult BMI results are easy to interpret; a BMI between 25 and 30 is considered overweight and a BMI of 30 is considered obese. BMI results for children (up to the age of 19) must also consider gender and age of the child in order to figure a percentile ranking. This BMI percentile ranking can determine if a child is underweight, at a healthy weight or at risk of being overweight.

◎ TIME
20 minutes

◎ MATERIALS
Bathroom scale
Yardstick
Pencil and paper
Calculator (optional)
BMI for Age Growth Chart for children
(available at www.cdc.gov)

◎ DIRECTIONS
1. Weight yourself on a bathroom scale. Record the result on paper.
2. Measure your height in inches. Record the result on paper. Be very accurate.
3. Using the following formula, calculate your BMI.

$$BMI = \frac{[your\ weight] \times 703}{height\ squared\ (height \times height)}$$

(BMI = weight divided by height squared x 703)

4. For children up to 19 years old, plot the results on the BMI for Age Growth Chart to obtain a percentile ranking.

◎ TECHNOLOGY ALTERNATE

1. Follow steps 1 and 2, above.
2. Use an online calculator to measure your BMI.

4. Dissect Food Labels

Learning to read food labels is important because it helps you to make better food choices, which is necessary to stay healthy. Learning to read and interpret food labels gives you the knowledge to select healthy foods and the appropriate size portions for good eating.

⊚ TIME
30 minutes

⊚ MATERIALS
Food labels from five different foods
Highlighter markers in five colors

⊚ DIRECTIONS
1. Collect five food labels from food that you recently consumed.
2. Discuss the information found on the USDA required food labels.
3. Using highlighter markers, highlight in the following way:
   • Serving size and calories: blue
   • Protein: green
   • Fiber: purple
   • Total fat: yellow
   • Sodium: pink
4. Discuss how to use this information to make healthy food choices.

⊚ TECHNOLOGY ALTERNATE
1. Use the Internet to explore food labels.
2. Create and print out a word search using words found on food labels.
3. Share the puzzle with family members and ask them to complete it.

5. Discover the Dietary Needs of Birds Native to Your Area

The inhabitants of nature have food and exercise requirements to stay healthy. Birds, the inhabitants we see on a daily basis, must have a balanced diet. This diet varies from species to species. Creating bird snacks can help birds maintain a healthy diet during months when food is scarce.

◎ TIME
30-minute sessions (2 sessions)

◎ MATERIALS
Guest speaker (from a bird watching group, aviary, or a veterinarian)
Recipe for a bird snack or homemade bird food
Ingredients and equipment to prepare recipe

◎ DIRECTIONS
Session 1:
1. Collect information about birds in your area.
2. List dietary needs for a balanced diet for these birds.
3. Discuss foods that are toxic to birds.
4. Research and find an easy recipe to make a bird snack or homemade bird food.

Session 2:
1. Assemble ingredients and equipment for recipe.
2. Prepare recipe.
3. Clean up work area.
4. Distribute bird snacks to participants for backyard use.

◎ TECHNOLOGY ALTERNATE
1. Collect information about birds from the Internet.
2. Create a pamphlet to illustrate dietary needs of birds found in your area.
3. Include an easy recipe for a bird snack or homemade bird food.
4. Share your completed pamphlet with others.

6. Go Beyond Food to Make a Meal Complete

Food is not the only component of a healthy meal. Using the correct size plates, bowls and glasses helps to control how much we eat. Sitting and enjoying our meals with others at a lovely, well-set table creates a pleasant atmosphere and stimulates conversation. This all contributes to eating smaller amounts and aids in digestion. The simple folding of a napkin is an easy, quick and inexpensive way to add interest to a table presentation.

⊙ TIME
40 minutes

⊙ MATERIALS
Cookbooks, magazines, family recipes
Utensils, dishes, bowls, glasses for serving
Paper or cloth napkins
Index cards and markers

⊙ DIRECTIONS
1. Discuss the three components of a meal: food, conversation and atmosphere.
2. Select a healthy lunch menu.
3. Select utensils, plates, bowls and glasses needed to serve the meal. Demonstrate how to correctly set the table.
4. Practice the art of creative napkin-folding (in shapes such as a candle, fleur-de-lis or sailboat).
5. To stimulate conversation, write some trivia questions on index cards about the foods you selected.

⊙ TECHNOLOGY ALTERNATE
1. Explore the three components of a meal online.
2. Practice napkin-folding by following online directions.

7. Test Your "Portion" Knowledge

Staying healthy involves not only eating the right foods but the right portion sizes. Portion size can be a problem nowadays. The diameter of plates, bowls and glasses has increased and the packaging of products has changed. Restaurants serve bigger portions on larger plates. Beverages are served in larger glasses and cups, as well. Fast food restaurants' supersizing of meals has created "portion distortion." Having some knowledge of correct portion sizes will go a long way in helping create healthy eating habits.

○ **TIME**

40 minutes

○ **MATERIALS**

Measuring equipment
Food and beverages such as pasta, vegetables, fruit, meat,
    cereal, cheese, lemonade
Portion size information guide
Golf ball, tennis ball, deck of cards, computer mouse, music CD
Healthy snacks (such as pretzels) for the winning team
A 10-inch plate, a six-inch bowl and eight-ounce glass

○ **DIRECTIONS**

1. Form two teams.
2. Have each team measure out what they think is a portion size of a selected food.
3. Check measurements with portion size information guide.
4. Discuss the results.
5. Record a point for the team that is correct.
6. Select an item such as a golf ball or deck of cards to match the correct portion size. (Use of these items, in the future, can help in selecting correct portion sizes when eating.)
7. Treat the winning team to a healthy snack.
8. Discuss the importance of using correct plate, bowl and glass sizes for healthy eating. Discuss how dining out affects portion size.

◎ **TECHNOLOGY ALTERNATE**

1. Search for pictures of foods online that represent correct portion size. (A good site to learn more about portion sizes is www.mypyramid.gov)
2. Create an online quiz to share with others that tests everyone's knowledge of healthy portion sizes.

Note to parents or staff utilizing this exercise. As an alternative to this exercise, choose a fast food restaurant that has nutritional information available online or in a handout at the counter. Ask participants to select their meal of choice and then ask for a "super-size" version of this meal. Have participants estimate how many times a week they eat fast food; then using their nutritional handouts, ask them to tabulate how many calories they are consuming with each meal, each week, and throughout the year (x 52). Ultimately, how many pounds (each pound equals 3,500 unused calories) would this eating pattern incur over a year's time?

8. Plant an Herb Garden

Gardening for the purpose of having fresh foods available can be rewarding and healthy. Planting an herb can be a good introduction to the gardening process. Harvested herbs can be used in recipes and shared with others in healthy food preparation.

◎ **TIME**

20 minutes

◎ **MATERIALS**

Container
Potting soil
Gardening tools
Seeds
Pocket diary

◎ **DIRECTIONS**

1. Discuss the responsibility and rewards of growing a garden.
2. Place potting soil in container.
3. Select an herb to grow and follow the package directions to plant seeds.
4. Water the planted seeds.
5. Write about the experience and keep a daily log.
6. Explore how to use the herb in healthy food preparation.
7. Harvest the herb when ready and use it in a recipe. Share your harvest with others.
8. Expand your garden with other plants or participate in a community garden project.

◎ **TECHNOLOGY ALTERNATE**

1. Plant seeds and use a camera to record the growing process.
2. Create an album to share with others.
3. Learn more about planting a garden through the Cooperative Extension System at www.extension.org/horticulture.

9. Take a "Popcorn Journey" from Farm to Bowl

Foods sold in today's grocery stores are often products of mass-production. Did you ever wonder what a certain food looked like before it was processed and packaged? Having some understanding of the journey a food takes from farm to table can lead to healthier eating habits.

◎ TIME

30 to 40 minutes

◎ MATERIALS

Popcorn on the cob
Package of popcorn (not microwave variety)
Popcorn popper (air popper or stovetop variety)
Vegetable oil
Preparation utensils and serving equipment
History and information about popcorn

◎ DIRECTIONS

1. Discuss history of popcorn, how and where it is grown and what makes it pop.
2. Let everyone touch and feel some popcorn before it is popped.
3. Select participants to help prepare the popcorn.
4. Pop the popcorn, observing the changes that take place.
5. Serve the popcorn.
6. Discuss why it is a nutritious snack; also discuss portion size and variations that can be made.
7. Read about the journey that popcorn takes from farm to table.
8. Explore the journeys that other snack foods take from farm to table.

◎ TECHNOLOGY ALTERNATE

1. Create a game with popcorn as the focus using a variety of technology mediums.

10. Build a "Run Through the Garden" Plan with a Buddy

Making changes in food choices, eating habits and daily exercise can be challenging. Successful changes can be rewarding and a healthier you can result. Planning and working on this with a friend can make the journey a more pleasant one. A friend can encourage, motivate, listen when you feel challenged and support you during this process. At the end, you and your friend can have fun celebrating your successes together.

◎ TIME
30 minutes for chart/plan
5 minutes each day to record results

◎ MATERIALS
Poster board
Yardstick or ruler
Markers, black and two colors
Pedometer (optional)

◎ DIRECTIONS
1. Select a friend to work with.
2. Using the poster board and black marker, create a scorecard to record your plan and its results. Scorecard categories should include: date, new food eaten, daily exercise time, eating habit change and TV/computer/video time.
3. Share ideas with your friend about how to complete the plan. Include new foods to taste or add to your diet, new activities to enjoy the outdoors and increase exercise (such as step counting), small changes to improve your eating habits and ways to manage TV/computer/video time.
4. Encourage, motivate, listen and support each other to carry out this plan.
5. Record results on chart on a regular basis, each one using a different color marker.
6. After a set amount of time, discuss the successes of your plan. Explore how you can improve.
7. Have fun and celebrate your success.

⊙ TECHNOLOGY ALTERNATE

1. Create a plan with a friend and use technology to carry out the plan.

Note to parents or staff utilizing this exercise. With this exercise, it is a good idea to be specific with possibly three goals in mind to be more healthy: losing weight by 1) cutting back or eliminating sugared drinks, 2) cutting back on snacks and 3) increasing exercise. Use specific goals that could be met through the benefits of a buddy system. Choose a reward to give participants at the end for their success in meeting their goals.

BIBLIOGRAPHY

Thousands of books, documentaries, research papers, web sites and news articles today express the urgent need to address the epidemic of childhood obesity. This list is limited to sources that inspired the author during his research for this book.

Alliance for a Healthier Generation, www.healthiergeneration.org.

American Obesity Association, www.obesity.org

Andrews, Ted. *Animal-Speak: The Spiritual and Magical Powers of Creatures Great and Small.* Llewellyn Publications, 12th Printing, 1997.

Barnard, Neal, MD. *Food for Life: How the New Four Food Groups Can Save Your Life.* Three Rivers Press, 1993.

Berg, Frances M. *Underage and Overweight: America's Childhood Obesity Crisis—What Every Family Needs to Know.* Hatherleigh Press, 2003.

Centers for Disease Control, www.cdc.gov.

Cooper, Alan. *The Inmates are Running the Asylum: Why High Tech Products Drive Us Crazy and How to Restore the Sanity.* Sams-Pearson Education, 2004.

Critser, Greg. *Fat Land: How Americans Became the Fattest People in the World.* Mariner Books, 2004.

Dalton, Sharron. *Our Overweight Children: What Parents, Schools and Communities Can Do to Control the Fatness Epidemic.* University of California Press, 2005.

Engel, Cindy. *Wild Health: Lessons in Natural Wellness from the Animal Kingdom.* Mariner Books, 2003.

Institute of Medicine of the National Academies. *Preventing Childhood Obesity: Health in the Balance.* National Academies Press, 2005.

Okie, Susan, MD. *Fed Up! Winning the War Against Childhood Obesity.* Joseph Henry Press, 2006.

Schlosser, Eric. *Fast Food Nation: The Dark Side of the All-American Meal.* Harper Perennial, 2005.

Spurlock, Morgan (writer and director). *Super Size Me.* 2004

Stein, Mathew. *When Technology Fails: A Manual for Self-Reliance, Sustainability and Surviving the Long Emergency.* Chelsea Green Publishing; 2nd edition, 2008.

Teachman, Bethany A., PhD; Schwartz, Marlene B., PhD; Gordic, Bonnie S.; Coyle, Brenda S., PhD. *Helping Your Child Overcome an Eating Disorder: What You Can Do at Home.* New Harbinger Publications, Inc., 2003.

United States Department of Agriculture, www.mypyramid.gov.

Weber, Karl; Participant Media. *Food Inc.: How Industrial Food is Making Us Sicker, Fatter, and Poorer—And What You Can Do About It.* PublicAffairs, media tie-in to the documentary, 2009.

Wilson, Charles; Schlosser, Eric. *Chew on This: Everything You Don't Want to Know About Fast Food.* Houghton Mifflin, 2007.

About the Author

꧁꧂

As a free-spirited boy who grew up during the Eisenhower administration, Roger Hall would run home from school, throw his books on the table and high-tail it outside to climb trees and play tag football. Now, as an older adult, Roger is deeply dismayed at the epidemic of childhood obesity in the United States. His heartfelt mission is to inspire today's youth to step away from technology, get outside and be in nature.

With more than 30 years in executive marketing, both domestic and international, Roger is a proven planner and strategist in market development and new product launches, and has consistently led organizations to substantial growth and profitability. Roger is the founding partner of Porcupine Communications.

Made in the USA
Charleston, SC
24 July 2011